Intermittent Fasting for Women

Faster Fat Loss

What You need to Know About Fasting

By Jessica Ward and Jon Peterson

Contents

Introduction   1

Chapter 1 Demystifying Intermittent Fasting   4

Chapter 2 Benefits Of Intermittent Fasting   16

Chapter 3 Intermittent Fasting For Women   28

Chapter 4 Techniques Of Intermittent Fasting   43

Chapter 5 Intermittent Fasting And Exercise   72

Chapter 6 Safety Tips For Women   79

Chapter 7 Tips To Stay Motivated   87

Chapter 8 The Biggest Mistakes To Avoid   95

Other Books By Author   100

Resources   101

Introduction

Most women who are unhappy with their body size want to lose some weight. Of course, some want to lose much more than others. The weight loss industry is filled with different strategies that are designed to help you shed those pounds. However, many women still struggle with getting rid of excess fat, and it can be very frustrating when you simply don't know what to do about it. The truth is that many of the popular strategies that are out there don't really cater to the specific needs of women. They have been designed with men in mind, and this is one of the reasons why most women end up unsatisfied with the results they see.

This book, *"Intermittent Fasting for Women: Faster Fat Loss,"* is written specifically with women in mind. Intermittent fasting has a lot of benefits for both men and women, but the main focus will be on helping women get the most out of this method. The bodies of men and women tend to respond differently when subjected to the fasting routine, and if you are not aware of this, you may find it difficult to attain any reasonable fat loss.

Intermittent fasting is totally natural. Your body is actually designed to work very efficiently with cycles of feasting and fasting. The problem we face today is a society where we simply have too much food available. We simply consume everything we see whenever we feel like it. The results speak for themselves. Almost 70% of Americans are overweight or obese, yet only 36% of this group actually accept that they have a weight problem! You are reading this book because you want to change the way your body looks, and intermittent fasting will help you do that.

You are going to learn what intermittent fasting really is and how it is different from your traditional dieting methods. Yes, there is a reason why conventional dieting methods don't work. We will also look at the many benefits of intermittent fasting, right before we dive into the different methods that you can use.

You will also learn how intermittent fasting affects women and what you need to do make sure that it works for you. There are some critical factors you need to consider if you want to ensure faster and effective fat loss. Exercise is also an important part of any weight loss program, so be prepared to learn some tips on how you, as a woman, can use it to lose weight. There are specific mistakes that most people make when fasting, and we will go through the major ones just to make sure you avoid some common pitfalls.

This book is a simple yet definitive guide to losing fat through intermittent fasting. Once you get used to the fasting cycles, you will start to see changes in your body that you never dreamed possible!

Chapter 1

Demystifying Intermittent Fasting

When you mention the word "fasting" to anyone today, the response is usually negative. Most people treat fasting as if it is some alien practice, yet the truth is that fasting isn't new at all. In fact, humans have been fasting intermittently for thousands of years.

Back when our ancestors used to run around hunting and gathering food, they would go for days without eating. Once they had managed to find, chase down, and kill their prey, they would carry the animal back home and feast on it. They wouldn't eat the whole thing at once. They would only consume small portions of food at specific times because they had no idea when or whether they would be successful in catching their next meal. According to the Salt Institute in California, our hunter-gatherer ancestors actually ate intermittently.

Today, thanks to modern technology, we don't have to live that way. We can get our food on demand without getting off the couch. Combine this with lack of adequate body exercise, and it's no wonder obesity is an epidemic. We have lost control of how much we eat and now consider fasting to be the preserve of the poor and sick.

So how does all this relate to intermittent fasting?

What is Intermittent Fasting?

Intermittent fasting is a pattern of eating where you allocate specific hours in a day for eating and spend the rest of the day abstaining from food. You fast for a specific number of hours and then consume all your daily calories within a specific window of time. This can also be done on a weekly cycle where you have days of fasting and days for eating normally. It is essentially a way of cycling through your feasting and fasting periods.

Here is a simple example of intermittent fasting. You eat your dinner by 7 pm in the evening and then go to bed. When you wake up, you don't eat any breakfast. You wait until around 10 am before you eat anything. The period between 7 pm and 10 am is your fasting window.

You are then allowed to eat anything you want between 10 am and 7 pm that evening. This is known as your "feasting" window. If you choose to exercise, you can do so before you begin your feasting period. It is important to note that during your fasting period, you can drink water and consume non-caloric beverages. Anything that contains sugar or alcohol should definitely be avoided.

As you can see, there are no major complications like having to drastically change your diet or eat lettuce all day. All you are required to do is stick to the feasting window you have chosen. You are the one who gets to choose the timings of your feasting and fasting windows. This adds to the flexibility of this technique.

History of Fasting

As we have discussed earlier, our ancestors practiced intermittent fasting due to the scarcity of food. There were times when they had a lot to eat and feasted on an animal they had killed. However, there were also many occasions where they had to get by on berries when food was scarce.

As civilizations progressed, mankind embraced religion and spirituality. Most religions encourage their members to fast during certain days purely for spiritual reasons. Written accounts from as far back as 200 AD reveal that fasting was used as a way of treating disease. A Greek philosopher called Plotinus once recommended to a Roman senator that he should fast on alternate days as a way to cure his gout. It is recorded that the senator's health improved and his condition disappeared. Ancient texts also suggest that philosophers like Hippocrates and Plato used to practice fasting as a way of improving their mental clarity and healing their bodies.

It is surprising to learn just how more in sync with their bodies people were back then compared to the people of today. They knew that fasting was good for the mind, body, and soul. Surprisingly enough, these are things your fancy, modern doctor won't tell you. If they did, how would they manage to sell millions of dollars worth of drugs for Big Pharma? Throughout history, we can see that ancient humans understood that consuming too much food on a regular basis causes disease.

Changing Your Mindset

But is intermittent fasting really natural?

Most people are sometimes concerned about having to go without food for extended periods of time. There is no need to worry about this. Fasting in this manner isn't unnatural. We normally spend many hours not eating anyway. A good example is when we are sleeping. So, in reality, every single person who sleeps through the night is actually fasting. This means there is no excuse you can give for not being able to stay away from food for a few hours a day. Intermittent fasting simply extends the amount of time that you go without food so that you can enjoy the fat loss benefits.

The problem is that we have believed the lie that our bodies need food at all times. As a result, we view fasting as some sort of starvation. We associate it with pain and end up gobbling up snacks thinking that we need all that food. If you want to embrace intermittent fasting and lose fat quickly, you must change your mindset.

Have you ever fallen sick at any time of your life? If you're like most normal people, then you definitely have. Have you ever wondered why when you get sick, you suddenly lose your appetite? The reason for that is simple. Your body is trying to inform you that you should abstain from eating too much so that it can have time to fight the disease and repair any damaged cells. Eliminating disease from the body requires energy, and digestion is one process that demands a lot of energy.

Your body cannot function effectively if it is always being forced to digest food. It needs time and energy to heal and repair the damage caused by the vagaries of everyday life. By fasting, you don't weaken your body. You make it stronger! Hormonal imbalances and genetic abnormalities are fixed; cells are repaired; insulin and blood sugar levels drop; your metabolism gets a boost, and your gut takes a break to heal. All these seemingly minor improvements are what ultimately bring about fat loss!

By practicing intermittent fasting, your body moves from burning glucose to burning fat to produce energy. Intermittent fasting on its own works wonders for your health. Now imagine what would happen if you added some light exercises. You would accelerate the fat-burning process and lose weight much faster!

Intermittent Fasting Versus Dieting

It is amazing just how many diets exist today. Every media source you turn to is hyping one type of diet or another. Most people insist that diets work, but if that was true, why are we not seeing tangible results on the ground? Women tend to form the largest group of people who are targeted by these diets, yet they are also the most frustrated by their failure to lose weight. Why are all the promises made by fitness gurus and health experts not bearing tangible and permanent results?

Here are a few points to ponder when contrasting dieting with intermittent fasting:

- The truth is that dieting is not natural. Contrary to public perception, dieting is purely an unnatural and quick-fix solution to a deeper problem. Most people who choose to go on a diet tend to have short-term goals. All they are interested in are the quick results. Think of it this way: how many people do you personally know who would want to diet for the rest of their life? That's right! Very few, if any at all! Dieting is disruptive to your regular routine, so nobody wants to be doing it forever. The moment you achieve that magic number on the weighing scale, your mind shifts and you subconsciously decide that you don't need the diet anymore. Pretty soon, you fall back into bad eating habits.

Intermittent fasting, on the other hand, is natural to humans. You make up your mind to eat only within a specific window and avoid consuming food the rest of the time. You don't have to change the foods you normally eat unless they are actively making you unhealthy. From a long-term perspective, maintaining intermittent fasting as a lifestyle is more sustainable.

- Almost all diets are structured in a way that recommends consuming food throughout the day. If the process of digestion itself consumes energy, and you are constantly filling your mouth with food, what happens to your body? You soon become trapped in a continuous energy-sapping loop! Yes, you are on a healthy diet, but you are still constantly tired and unable to lose any significant amount of body fat. However, intermittent fasting gives your body a break during the fasting period. All your eating and calorie-burning is scheduled within a small window of time. In fact, studies show that you can lose weight faster if you restrict your eating to a small window of time rather than eating many small meals throughout the day.

- Your regular diet plan tries to limit the amount of food you can eat per meal. This seems like a good idea, but how many people enjoy having to count calories accurately every time they get hungry? And if you somehow find it easy to do so, do you always have the self-discipline necessary to stick to the diet plan? How do you feel being restricted to particular types of foods and not others? These are all issues you won't have to deal with when fasting. Intermittent fasting allows you to eat whatever you want and whatever portions you decide, just as long as you can stick to your health and weight loss goals.

The point here is that most diet programs are unsustainable, restrictive, and stressful. Now you understand why many people start a diet, stop suddenly, and then start all over again. The body is fighting the unnatural eating system that has been forced upon it and is sabotaging the person's weight loss efforts. On the other hand, intermittent fasting is natural and the body isn't even forced to adapt. It is only your mind that requires a shift in thinking.

Differences in Men and Women

So far, we have been learning about intermittent fasting from a general perspective. However, it is about time we started drawing a line between how it affects women in contrast to men.

For men, there isn't much to worry about when it comes to fasting.

For women, on the other hand, there are specific factors that make things a little more complicated. Studies show that women must take care when fasting due to some reported side effects. There have been reports of irregular menstrual periods, changes in metabolism, and in some cases, early onset menopause. There are also certain categories of women who shouldn't practice intermittent fasting at all.

But this isn't meant to scare women away from practicing intermittent fasting. This is a way of letting you know that there is more information you need to learn about before you start. This book wants to teach you how to do it right. You need to learn how it will affect you, your weight loss, as well as your overall health. Before we go deeper into how women should practice intermittent fasting, let's look at some of its major benefits.

Chapter 2

Benefits of Intermittent Fasting

Intermittent fasting involves going for 12 or more hours without consuming anything except water. For those who have bought into the myth that you must eat six meals every day to keep your metabolism up, this can be a daunting task. However, science has proven that intermittent fasting actually has numerous benefits. These benefits are related to weight loss, muscle growth, cognitive function, and general health.

In this chapter, we are going to look at what intermittent fasting has to offer you.

Weight Loss Benefits

There are many diets out there that claim to provide weight loss benefits. Some recommend the elimination of certain food groups while others focus on reducing your portion sizes. You may have tried one of these diets before and lost a bit of weight. However, the majority of people have failed to lose weight in the long term.

What differentiates intermittent fasting from all the other diets is consistency. There is no special diet or unique meal plan. All you have to do is follow whatever meal plan you want and be consistent throughout (Read *IIFYM: The Ultimate Beginner's Guide*).

Most women who practice intermittent fasting will automatically consume fewer meals. It is important not to binge on food so that you don't end up increasing your calorie intake above normal.

A study conducted in 2012 revealed that intermittent fasting on its own (with no exercise) could lead to a 3% to 8% drop in weight in less than six months. The women who participated in the study reported that their waistlines shrank by 4% to 7%.

Here are some specific weight loss benefits:

1.   It boosts your metabolic rate

Studies show that staying in a fasted state leads to a spike in the hormone *norepinephrine*. This hormone increases your basal metabolic rate and burns fat. On top of that, once you enter your eating window, your metabolism still stays at an elevated level. You are essentially burning excess fat even when eating!

2.   Reduction of insulin levels in the bloodstream

When your insulin levels go down, so does your blood sugar. Your body is then forced to burn fat to produce energy. According to the US National Institutes of Health, a reduction in insulin can also elevate your metabolic rate by up to 14%.

This drop in insulin levels also triggers the increase in production of human growth hormone (HGH). This hormone increases your body's ability to convert fat into energy and also build more muscle. Women shouldn't worry about gaining too much muscle. You don't have enough testosterone to bulk up like the guys unless you work out like a wrestler and start popping steroids.

3. Less food consumption

One of the things you will notice over time is that you will begin to consume less food within your feasting window. Try to examine your food portions during your intermittent fast, and you'll see this clearly. Research shows that when fasting, you end up consuming 20% less food than the period before you began fasting. This is possibly due to the levels of the ghrelin hormone being normalized. Ghrelin is responsible for controlling appetite and triggering hunger, and in most of us, this hormone doesn't function efficiently. Due to our modern diet, a lot of our hormones are out of sync, which is why we feel hungry and eat all the time. Once your ghrelin starts working properly, you will feel less hungry.

Muscle Growth Benefits

The more muscle you have, the faster your metabolic rate. In other words, gaining muscle is another way to reduce fat in your body. Women shouldn't look at muscles as something only men are interested in. Even women can do with a bit of strength training occasionally, just to keep the body toned and fit.

Most people believe that fasting and muscle gain are incompatible. The misconception has always been that you need to be constantly eating enough protein to maintain lean muscle. If not, then your body will start feeding on your muscle tissue. However, this is not true. Just because you don't eat every few hours does not mean your muscles won't grow. The most important aspect of muscle growth is actually the quantity of food you eat every day.

There is only one condition under which your body would start breaking down muscle for energy. *This is if you go without food for longer than 24 straight hours.* This makes it highly unlikely that you would suffer muscle loss when practicing intermittent fasting the right way.

These are the benefits of intermittent fasting in relation to muscle growth:

1. Contrary to popular perception, fasting actually increases your energy levels over time. This means you can still squeeze out an effective workout even when fasting. The elevated energy levels are a result of increased mitochondrial energy. You need to know that in the early days of fasting, you will definitely feel a bit tired, but this condition will be reversed when your body finally adapts to the new eating schedule.

2. Fasting allows the body to rest, repair damaged cells, and eliminate any waste materials from the body. This is especially critical after a strenuous workout when the body needs to repair muscles and get rid of lactic acid.

3. Fasting boosts production of human growth hormone (HGH), which some refer to as the "fitness hormone." Research suggests that intermittent fasting can increase HGH levels up to five times the normal count. When this happens, your liver produces a protein (IGF-1) that triggers cell growth throughout your body. HGH is known to increase your ability to grow bigger muscles, strengthen bones, heal injuries, and stay fit. Some scientists also claim that IGF-1 has the ability to boost longevity.

Cognitive Benefits

These are the benefits of intermittent fasting on your brain:

1. It preserves your memory and learning functions. Research shows that fasting for 10 to 16 hours forces your body to break down fats into fatty acids known as ketones. When ketones enter the bloodstream, they protect your memory and learning capability. Some studies indicate that intermittent fasting has

the potential of boosting the memory of the elderly.

2. It boosts production of a protein known as brain neurotrophic growth factor. This protein protects neurons and stimulates their growth. This has the effect of improving your resilience to neurological stress, therefore preventing neurodegenerative diseases. Intermittent fasting also helps your body to eliminate damaged proteins from cells in the brain.

3. It stimulates changes in the genes that are linked to the healthy aging of your brain. These genes are also known to protect your brain from certain diseases.

General Health Benefits

According to researchers, intermittent fasting provides physiological benefits because it places your cells under some stress. This mild stress forces your body to adapt by increasing its ability to resist stress and diseases. In other words, you are training your body to withstand the harsh conditions and pressures of everyday life. This proves that it isn't always a bad thing when you place some stress on your body and mind.

Here are some of the general health benefits of intermittent fasting:

1. Lowering food consumption by 30% has been proven to reduce your risk of diabetes, inflammation, and heart disease.

2. It improves your cardiovascular health. Studies show that intermittent fasting boosts the levels of adiponectin in the bloodstream. This hormone prevents the formation of plaque on the walls of your arteries, thus minimizing the risk of ischemic injury to the heart.

3. It slows down the progression of cancer. A study conducted on mice at the Duke University Medical Center in North Carolina showed that the caloric deficit resulting from

intermittent fasting actually slowed down cancer in the mice.

4. It reduces the level of oxidative stress and inflammation in the body. In one study, participants who were overweight and had asthma were asked to practice intermittent fasting for eight weeks. Those who did so managed to lose 8% of their body weight and their asthma symptoms improved as well. It was also discovered that there was an improvement in a number of their quality-of-life indicators.

5. At a cellular level, intermittent fasting provides you with the same benefits as exercise. It helps your cells cope better with stress and slows down aging.

6. Studies show that intermittent fasting leads to an increase in productivity. Considering the fact that you don't have to focus on food all day, you will quickly learn that you become more productive during your fasting periods. There is

less concern with planning and cooking meals, and you end up saving money as well.

7. It reduces the level of lipids in your bloodstream. This includes a decrease in LDL cholesterol and triglycerides.

8. It causes changes in parasympathetic and sympathetic activity, which results in reduced blood pressure.

You need to understand that intermittent fasting is not a fad or quick fix to help you lose fat. It is more of a technique that focuses on moderation and lifestyle management. The benefits you have read about in this chapter can only be experienced if you practice intermittent fasting properly. One of the things to avoid is binge eating on your feast days.

If you set a weekly target for weight loss, make sure that you can maintain that target. Settle on something that you can achieve, for example, losing half a pound a week. Losing more than one pound a week will put you in trouble as you won't be able to sustain it for very long. Your weight loss progress will slow down and ultimately stagnate. Intermittent fasting is a lifestyle that advocates for consistency and sustainable weight management.

Now that you are aware of the numerous benefits of intermittent fasting let's look at how intermittent fasting affects women in particular.

Chapter 3

Intermittent Fasting for Women

Intermittent fasting offers numerous benefits for both men and women, especially in the areas of fat loss and overall health. However, women need to understand some of the factors that come into play. We all know that women's bodies are different from those of men, and in most cases, this doesn't matter. However, when it comes to intermittent fasting, such differences have an impact.

Most of the research conducted on intermittent fasting has not factored in the physiological differences between men and women. Some women have complained that they haven't experienced the positive results that men keep talking about. Women have reported symptoms such as mood swings, fatigue, hormone problems, and infertility.

Let's start by sharing the experience of a female medical doctor who has tried the fast and now understands how women should go about it.

The Experience

Dr. Amy Shah is a certified doctor who practices medicine in Phoenix, Arizona. She is certified in Internal Medicine and Allergy & Immunology. After learning of the potential benefits that intermittent fasting could have on women's health, she went ahead and tried it. According to Dr. Shah, the experience didn't go as she had expected the first time round. She knew that intermittent fasting was supposed to lead to clarity of mind and increased energy, but that was not how she felt.

On day one, she failed to eat enough food within her feasting window. That night, she didn't get much sleep due to the veracity of her hunger pangs. Naturally, she woke up exhausted and cranky. On day two, she decided to change tact and stuffed herself with food. After that, she started experiencing hunger and hormonal changes that she couldn't control at all. Within a mere seven days, Dr. Shah quit her fast.

Being the diligent doctor that she is, Dr. Shah started asking herself whether other women had experienced similar symptoms or whether what she had gone through was simply peculiar to her. After performing an internet search, she discovered that many other women had also complained about intermittent fasting and how it messed with their hormones.

She knew that if women were to enjoy the benefits that came with intermittent fasting, there had to be a way to resolve the hormonal challenges.

You and Your Hormones

The truth is that intermittent fasting can result in a hormonal imbalance in the body of a woman if the appropriate steps are not followed. Women's bodies are much more sensitive to the signals of starvation compared to those of men. Women have reproductive cycles that are very specific and precisely-timed. Men don't really have cycles to worry about, and the timing of their reproduction isn't as precise. This means that women have to be more careful.

Researchers from the Department of Biotechnology at the Guru Nanak Dev University in India conducted a study on male and female rats. Their aim was to study the effects of intermittent fasting on the reproductive health of animals. After three months of testing, the results showed that intermittent fasting caused a significant drop in body weight and blood glucose in both the male and female rats. The female rats had lost 19% of their body weight while the male rats had shed 34% of their weight.

However, the fasting also affected the Luteinizing Hormone in the female rats. The ovaries of the female rats had reduced in size, and this interrupted their menstrual cycle. It also induced more insomnia in the female rats than it did in the males. To be honest, though, the male rats also experienced a reduction in testosterone production. The control group of female rats, on the other hand, showed a regular ovulation and estrous cycle.

The conclusion of this study proved that when food is scarce, an animal will adjust its energy requirements and invest more in survival than reproduction. When there isn't enough food in the body to sustain your metabolic needs, you can experience delayed puberty, as well as suppression of ovulation and menstrual cycle.

So, what does this mean for you?

As a woman, when your body senses starvation, it triggers a massive increase in the two hunger hormones – *Ghrelin* and *Leptin*. Since you will be consuming less food during your feasting window than you normally would on a regular day, production of these hormones is ramped up further. This causes you to feel an insatiable hunger. Research indicates that this insatiable hunger that a woman feels is actually a way for the female body to protect a potential fetus. It doesn't matter if you are pregnant or not. The hormones are designed to warn you that you aren't getting enough food and you should eat more.

Now, if you are a woman who is trying to lose weight, you are obviously going to ignore these hunger pangs. You will choose to wait for your eating window before you eat anything. This will simply cause more hunger hormones to be released. The worst case scenario is where you succumb to the pressure and then binge during your eating window. You then feel guilty and end up under-eating the next time, leading to starvation again. It is this vicious cycle that ultimately interrupts the normal functioning of your hormones and even prevents ovulation.

Unfortunately, there aren't many studies that have been done on humans to explore how intermittent fasting affects women compared to men. Even though the studies mentioned above were performed on rats, they show the effects of intermittent fasting on the female body. There is potential for hormonal imbalances, fertility problems, fatigue, bloating, headaches, and insomnia. There is also the possibility that it may worsen eating disorders such as bulimia and anorexia.

So, what now? Do you give up on intermittent fasting as a solution to your weight problems? No! There is a solution!

Crescendo Fasting

There a number of options available, but the best way for a woman to practice intermittent fasting is through the Crescendo method. What you need to realize with intermittent fasting is that you will only get into trouble if you dive into it too quickly. This applies more to those people who are new to fasting. For this reason, it is important to modify the intermittent fasting routine.

The most popular method of intermittent fasting is the 16/8 method, where you fast every day for 16 hours and only eat within an eight-hour period. Crescendo fasting is where you only fast for a number of days in a week rather than doing it every day. You fast for only two or three days a week, and keep your fasting window to about 12 – 16 hours. Don't fast for consecutive days! Make sure that you alternate your fasting days.

This will help you gradually ease into the fasting routine without negatively affecting your hormones. Your body will have enough time to adapt to the new eating schedule and still enjoy the same benefits of intermittent fasting. If you practice Crescendo fasting the right way, you will lose body fat, gain energy, and boost your inflammatory markers.

Rules to Follow:

1. Fast for two or three days a week, on alternating days - For example, you can decide to fast on Monday, Wednesday, and Friday. Alternatively, you can fast on Tuesday, Thursday, and Saturday. The most important

thing is to ensure that you have an eating window between every two fasting days.

2. Maintain a fasting window of about 12 to 16 hours - In case you are fasting for the first time, make sure that you start with the minimum number of hours and work your way up. When in a fasted state, you can engage in light strength exercises and some cardio.

3. On your feasting days, make sure you eat as normal - Since you aren't fasting on these days, you can schedule some HIIT (high-intensity interval training) exercises. You can spend one or more hours engaging in intense exercises such as running or biking.

4. Get enough water to drink - Always make sure that you drink enough water when fasting. You also have the option of consuming black tea and black coffee, but don't add any sweeteners or milk.

5. Follow this routine for two weeks - After you get used to this cycle, you can then add an extra day of fasting.

6. It is recommended that you take between five and eight grams of BCAAs when fasting - This is optional, but these branched chain amino acid supplements don't have many calories and can give your muscles the necessary fuel. This will help reduce the intensity of the fatigue and hunger pangs. It is also recommended that you take your BCAAs in powder rather than tablet form. Tablets may be less expensive, but they are more of a hassle.

If you want to gauge how your body will respond to fasting, you can also decide to do a trial fast. You get to learn more about your hunger signals and hormonal reactions without necessarily committing to anything. A trial fast is only done for one day. You can fast for a couple of hours or decide to go a full 24 hours without food. For example, you can have your breakfast at 8 am and spend the entire day without food. The next meal will come at 8 am the following day. You can drink water, tea, and engage in some light exercises. It is also important to plan your meals in advance so that you aren't driven to make unhealthy diet choices when hungry.

What to Eat

You may be wondering what kinds of foods to consume during your eating window. Intermittent fasting doesn't really recommend that you abandon certain foods and replace them with others. However, since you do want to lose weight without harming your hormonal balance, some food items can help.

1. Nuts and legumes – These are a good source of fats. They contain the good kind of cholesterol and provide enough energy to keep you going when you are fasting. Legumes and nuts also contain folate, which is a mineral that boosts your reproductive health. Nuts such as macadamia, peanuts, and pecan are great for

alleviating any cravings you may have, especially during that first week. Avoid carb-heavy foods because though they leave your stomach full, they don't provide long-lasting energy.

2. Seeds – Flax, pumpkin, and sunflower seeds are a great option when trying to lose weight.

3. Proteins – It is important to consume some animal protein as well as from plant sources. Poultry and fish should be part of your diet at least three times a week.

4. Kale – You should consider complementing your meals with kale. This vegetable contains protein and is a rich source of iron, magnesium, and vitamin B. Iron performs a similar function to folate, so you can skip legumes on some days and eat kale.

5. Fruits – They are loaded with the vitamins and minerals you require for good health. They also keep you full and energetic for longer periods.

When to Stop Fasting

There are specific signs and symptoms that you need to watch out for when practicing intermittent fasting. Of course, if you do it right and follow the Crescendo method, you will be on the safe side. However, stop fasting if you start experiencing the following:

- Irregular periods

- Extreme lethargy

- Acne and other skin conditions

- Irregular sleeping patterns

- Mood swings or depression

- Sluggish immune system

- Reduced sex drive

- Poor muscle recovery

- Poor digestion (bloating)

Women Who Shouldn't Fast

There are certain categories of women who are advised against any form of fasting. These include:

- Pregnant women – Though you may feel that you need to do something about the added weight, it is not recommended that you fast while pregnant. You may risk your health and the pregnancy. Just keep eating according to your body's needs.

- Women with a history of eating disorders, for example, anorexia or bulimia.

- Women who are chronically depressed and stressed – Fasting tends to add extra stress on the body. This is something you don't need when you are feeling low and tired.

- Women who are struggling with irregular sleeping patterns.

- Women who are on medication

- Women who suffer from low blood pressure

Intermittent fasting provides numerous benefits to the body, and there is no reason why women should be left out because of their biological and physiological makeup. As long as you do it the smart way, you too will reap all the benefits and minimize the risks. Just eat healthy foods, exercise a little and watch out for any of the warning signs mentioned. The guidelines provided here will help you start well and safely maintain your fasting.

Chapter 4

Techniques of Intermittent Fasting

When it comes to intermittent fasting, there are many variations to choose from. Unlike many other regular diets that have only one fixed way of doing things, intermittent fasting is very flexible and allows you to choose how you want to practice it. This level of customization is one of the aspects that make intermittent fasting so popular.

So, what does this mean for you?

People tend to react differently when placed under the same fasting technique. This means that if a fasting technique worked for one person, it doesn't necessarily mean that you will be comfortable with it. As an individual, it is important that you find the intermittent fasting technique that best fits your situation. It is usually a good idea to try the different techniques to get a feel of them.

In this chapter, we cover the most popular intermittent fasting techniques. They are all effective for fat loss and improving your general health and fitness. However, as a woman, keep in mind what you have learned in the previous chapter. This will help you settle on a technique that is safe and suitable for you.

The 16/8 Protocol

This is one of the more popular ways of practicing intermittent fasting. It is also known as the *Leangains Protocol.* It is called 16/8 because it recommends 16 hours of fasting and allocates 8 hours for your eating window. Most people would view the 8-hour eating window as being too short, but it is actually possible to fit three good meals within this time frame.

One of the great things about the 16/8 protocol is that you can schedule your fasting window to include the time you spend sleeping. Once you have taken your dinner, you simply avoid eating any dessert and go to sleep. When you wake up, you skip breakfast and wait to eat at the scheduled time.

For example, let's say that you take your dinner at 7 pm in the evening. You go to sleep thereafter and on waking up in the morning, you only drink water and non-caloric beverages. Since you need to fast for 16 hours, your eating window will begin at 11 am.

The Leangains protocol was created specifically for professional body builders and athletes who needed to cut fat and build muscle at the same time. However, you don't have fall into these two categories to take advantage of the benefits of this technique. It is recommended that men fast for the full 16 hours while women fast for 14 hours. Research shows that female professional athletes tend to improve their performance if they fast for shorter periods of time.

One important thing to note about the 16/8 method is that you are required to stick to whole and unprocessed foods. If you plan on exercising often, you have to follow a balanced diet as much as possible. After heavy exercise, make sure that you consume more complex carbohydrates than fats. This is to help your body recover from the strenuous workout. On days where your exercise is light, eat more fats than carbohydrates. The only thing that you should maintain is your protein consumption level.

The 16/8 method is flexible with regard to the frequency of your meals within your feasting window. The only challenge you may have with it is the fact that it specifies the types of food to consume, especially if you are exercising. For some people, having to strictly follow an eating plan can be difficult.

Sample Setup of Leangains Protocol

Since Leangains is pretty flexible, there are different setups that you can follow. These setups are inclusive of workout sessions.

1. Fasted training

This is where you train before you begin your eating phase. In Chapter 3, one of the rules of Crescendo Fasting was taking BCAAs to provide fuel for your muscles and relieve hunger pangs. It is recommended that you consume about 8 grams of BCAAs as part of your "pre-workout meal," which shouldn't be counted as part of your feeding window. You can mix the BCAA powder into a shake and drink it five to fifteen minutes before your workout.

9 pm – Final meal before your fast

11:30 to 12 am – Pre-workout meal of 8 grams BCAA

12 to 1 pm – Exercise

1 pm – First and largest (post-workout) meal of the day

4 pm – Next meal

9 pm – Final meal before your fast

2. Morning fasted training

This will work well for you if you would rather exercise early in the day.

8 to 9 pm – Final meal before fast

6 am – 8 grams BCAA

6 to 7 am – Exercise

8 am – 8 grams BCAA

10 am – 8 grams BCAA

12 to 1 pm - First and largest (post-workout) meal of the day

8 to 9 pm – Final meal of the day

3. One pre-workout meal

For younger people who either have flexible hours or are in college, this setup may fit you better.

8 to 9 pm – Final meal before fast

12 to 1 pm – Pre-workout meal containing ¼ of your daily calorie intake

3 to 4 pm – Exercise

4 to 5 pm – Largest (post-workout) meal

8 to 9 pm – Final meal of the day

4. Two pre-workout meals

Some people work normal hours and can't squeeze in a workout early in the morning or in the middle of the afternoon. This setup might be suitable.

8 to 9 pm – Final meal before fast

12 to 1 pm – First meal containing ¼ of your daily calorie intake

4 to 5 pm – Pre-workout meal containing ¼ of your daily calorie intake

6 to 8 pm – Exercise

8 to 9 pm – Largest meal of the day

There is no need to overanalyze which of the above setups is better than the other. The important thing is to look at your daily behavioral patterns and go with the setup that suits you best. Each of the above setups has its own strengths and benefits.

It is also important that you learn to maintain a constant eating window, regardless of the setup that you choose to go with. This is because of hormonal entrainment of your feeding patterns. If you normally break your fast at 12 to 1 pm and your eating window closes at 9 pm, try to stick to that schedule throughout.

The 5:2 Diet

This technique is also referred to as the Fast Diet and was made popular by a British journalist and doctor called Michael Mosley. It recommends that you eat as you normally would for five days of the week and then reduce your calorie intake for two days in a week. Women are advised to consume no more than 500 calories on fasting days. For the men, 600 calories are recommended when fasting.

The name is a bit misleading since it isn't really your traditional diet but more of an eating pattern. This method is flexible because it allows you to choose which two days of the week you prefer to fast. As always, just make sure that they are not consecutive days. The 5:2 diet also doesn't hinder your food choices; only when you should eat them. You can split your calorie intake on fasting day into two meals. For women, this would mean 250 calories per meal.

It must be said that when we talk about "eating normally" on your non-fasting days, it doesn't mean that you should binge on your favorite junk food. Remember that your goal is to lose fat faster, so if you don't watch what you eat, you won't achieve it. The 5:2 diet is very effective for fat loss because it helps you consume fewer calories than you normally would. This is why you shouldn't try to compensate for your reduced calorie intake by bingeing on your regular eating days.

If you are the kind of person who must have breakfast, then you can budget your 500 calories by spreading them across three small meals. On the other hand, if you prefer to start eating later in the day, you can eat a big lunch and a dinner. It is recommended that you focus on eating more high-protein and high-fiber foods to keep you full.

So what kind of foods can help you stay satiated while allowing you to consume less than 500 calories a day? Here are a few good options:

- Soups – For example tomato, miso, vegetable, or cauliflower soup

- Natural yogurt plus berries

- Tea

- Black coffee

- Cauliflower Rice

- Boiled eggs

- Grilled lean meat or fish

These are just a few examples of foods you can eat. It is up to you to experiment and find out what is most suitable for you. There are a number of great resources to help you make a decision about how to eat according to the calories you need. You can check out *IIFYM: The Ultimate Beginner's Guide* if you want to lose weight and not give up your favorite foods.

Sample Fast Diet Meal Plans

Plan 1

Breakfast:

- 3.5 ounces natural low-fat yogurt – 65 calories

- 2 sweet plums – 60 calories

- 1 teaspoon honey – 20 calories

Dinner:

- 2 ounces tuna mayo – 171 calories

- Cracked black pepper – No calories

- 2 Ryvita cracker breads – 70 calories

- 2.5 ounces rocket sprinkled on top – 12 calories

Snack:

- Miso soup – 32 calories

Total daily calorie count - 430

Plan 2

Lunch: (Spanish omelet)

- 2 eggs – 140 calories

- 2 ½ ounces spinach leaves – 20 calories

- Salt and pepper – No calories

Dinner:

- 1 ½ ounces hummus – 123 calories

- Fill a medium-sized bowl with cucumber, raw pepper, and carrots – 52 calories

Snack:

- 2 ½ ounces Edamame beans with rock salt – 84 calories

Total daily calorie count – 419

Plan 3

Breakfast:

- 3 ½ ounces strawberries – 30 calories

- 3 ½ ounces blueberries – 57 calories

- 3 ½ ounces raspberries – 28 calories

Dinner: (Harissa chicken and grilled veggie couscous)

- 1 tablespoon harissa paste – 15 calories

- 3 ½ ounces veggie couscous – 139 calories

- ¼ pound chicken breast – 160 calories

Snack:

- 10 pistachios - 60 calories

Total daily calorie count – 489

Plan 4

Lunch:

- 1 soft boiled egg – 70 calories

- 5 asparagus pieces – 20 calories

- Season with salt and pepper

Dinner: (corn-on-the-cob and turkey burgers)

- 1 corn-on-the-cob – 156 calories

- 4 ounces of (turkey mince, a small egg, garlic, chili, and spring onion) – 172 calories

Snack:

- A couple of frozen grapes – 60 calories

Total daily calorie count – 478

Plan 5

Breakfast:

- 2 egg omelets with 2 ounces red pepper and 2 ounces onions – 156 calories

Lunch:

- 1 sachet miso soup – 14 calories
- 2 carrot sticks – 50 calories

Dinner:

- Small sirloin steak with 7 ounces of mixed lettuce salad, drizzled with lemon – 275 calories

Total daily calorie count - 495

The Eat-Stop-Eat Method

This is a technique that involves fasting for a whole 24 hours for one or two days of the week. This type of intermittent fasting is chosen by people whose diets are already healthy, but they simply desire to boost their well-being.

It is an extremely flexible method. There are no specified eating windows, and you can eat at any time on your eating days. If you decide to eat normally on Monday, then you must spend the whole of Tuesday without food. So, if your last meal was dinner on Monday, your next meal should be dinner on Tuesday. You can continue with your normal eating schedule for Wednesday and Thursday, and then fast on Friday. Keep in mind that the daily calorie intake for women is generally 2,000 calories. The above is just an example to get you to understand the eat-stop-eat method. How you pick your fasting days within the week is up to you. It shouldn't be a problem fitting it into your daily schedule.

Unlike the 5:2 diet, there are no calorie restrictions here. Just keep it to a maximum of two days of fasting per week, and don't fast on consecutive days. Also, make sure to stay hydrated when fasting by drinking enough water and non-alcoholic drinks (tea or coffee). In case you want to lose fat and tone your muscles as well, it is recommended that you engage in some resistance training. For your non-fasting days, it is also recommended that you eat a lot of fruits, veggies, and spices.

Fasting for a full 24 hours can be difficult for most people, especially if you have never tried it before. As we discussed before, to avoid complications, just begin with a 14 hour fast for two days of the week. Once you get adjusted to it, you can start increasing your fasting window. As always, do not binge on your normal days. Since this method doesn't have any kind of specified meal plan, it is up to you to determine what to eat. You are aiming for fat loss, so have the self-control and discipline required to stick to a diet that aligns with your goals.

The Alternate-Day Diet

This method is exactly as the name describes. You diet for one day, eat normally the next, and diet the day after that. It isn't really a total fast. On the days that you diet, you are required to slash your calorie intake down to a $1/5^{th}$ of what you normally consume. For example, if your average daily intake is 2,000 calories, you should consume 400 calories on your fasting days. Your fasting days are called "Down Days" while your normal eating days are referred to as "Up Days." This is why it is also referred to as the UpDayDownDay Diet.

There is the risk of exceeding your calorie intake on your Down Days. To avoid such a scenario, the Alternate-Day Diet recommends that you consume liquid foods instead of solid ones. In other words, you should prepare replacement shakes containing essential nutrients and sip them throughout the day. This is only a strategy to get you through the initial two weeks of this diet. After that, you can revert back to consuming solid foods.

On your Up Days, you should try to get as much intense exercise as possible to cut down on body fat. As always, try not to binge on these days and create a strict meal plan to help you stay on course.

This fasting technique is designed for people who have a high level of self-discipline and have a specific weight target that they want to achieve. While some people may find it suitable, others may not be comfortable with it. Here are some pros and cons of alternate-day fasting.

Pros:

1. It helps cut body fat – This technique can be quite effective in helping you lose fat and shed a couple of pounds. In fact, research shows that Alternate-Day Fasting is more effective in

lowering your fat mass compared to a strict calorie reduction diet. This is good news for those who are obese.

2. It helps to prevent chronic diseases – Both animal and human trials have proved that the Alternate-Day Diet can prevent cancer, cardiovascular disease, and diabetes.

3. It is easier to follow than your traditional dieting routine – Dieting can be hard. This is especially true if you are forced to count calories every day and are restricted to specific foods. Most people quit after a few weeks of dieting because of all the restrictions you have to deal with daily. However, the guidelines for the Alternate-Day Diet are simple. Eat whatever you want on Up Days and minimize calorie intake on Down Days.

Cons:

1. Making a long-term commitment can be difficult – The study that compared the

Alternate-Day Diet and a strict calorie restriction diet showed some other interesting results. The group following this form of fasting had a higher dropout rate than the calorie restricting group. The alternate-day fasting participants that managed to stick it out till the end also slipped up more than the other group. Their biggest challenge was overeating on their Up Days. A different study even revealed that people who go on the Alternate-Day Diet tend to experience constant hunger on their Down Days, yet it is expected that hunger should recede with time. This technique may be suitable for losing fat quickly, but it isn't sustainable for the long term.

2. It leaves you too tired and hungry to work out – Down Days can be very difficult to handle, and hitting the gym may not be possible.

It is recommended that you talk to your physician before you embark on this type of fast. This is in case you are taking medication that needs to go with food. To avoid bingeing on your Up Days, you should also prepare a meal plan in advance. If you choose to try this method of intermittent fasting, just ease yourself into it to avoid stressing your mind and body.

The Warrior Diet

This form of intermittent fasting isn't for everyone. Going by the name itself, you should be able to tell that it involves some extreme discipline. The Warrior Diet involves spending about 20 hours in an under-eating phase, getting by on tiny portions of fruits, veggies, and protein. The only large meal you are allowed to consume is dinner, and you only have the remaining four hours to do this. This is not just any regular dinner, either. It must be whole and unprocessed foods or Paleo.

The Warrior Diet is founded on the principles of cutting edge science and evolutionary biology. It relies on research shows that human beings are naturally nocturnal eaters who are adapted to eating one large meal at the end of the day. This is something that modern society has abandoned, and today we eat too many meals at the wrong time of the day. The Warrior Diet aims to nourish your body according to two phases – daytime feeding and nighttime feeding. This ultimately shifts your metabolism toward burning rather than gaining body fat.

This technique works on the principle that your body will improve its performance when it is only allowed to feast within a four-hour window at night. The fruits, veggies, and protein are meant to keep your nervous system stimulated, energy levels up, and metabolism running. Don't forget that what you eat throughout the day are only small portions. So, save the overeating for the night feast. This may sound odd, but overindulging at night is actually encouraged, since it apparently improves digestion, boosts cell repair and calmness, and helps in healing the nervous system.

The Warrior Diet is also very strict in the way you are supposed to structure your dinner meals. You are restricted to eating your vegetables first, followed by proteins, and then fats. In case you are still not satisfied, you can then finish off with some nuts. Though you can eat a huge meal within the four hours, you are better off splitting your meal into different components. It doesn't really matter how much food you eat. Just try to listen to your body and stop when you feel full.

The truth is that this method of intermittent fasting is likely to mess with your social life. While you will be able to snack on a few things during the day, the stringent guidelines regarding the sequence of dinner are not sustainable in the long term. There aren't many people who would want to survive on snacks all day and binge at night before going to sleep. Doing this every day is a pretty tough thing to do, and that's why it is only for those who consider themselves warriors.

Here are some guidelines that can help you along the way:

1. Drink a lot of clean water – In the under-eating phase, try to drink as much filtered water as possible. The recommended daily amount is eight glasses, but this is a minimum number, so aim to exceed it. This should be taken more seriously on those days when you plan on working out, whether it is walking, running, or resistance training.

2. Eat enough protein – Since it is recommended that you eat small amounts of proteins during the day, make sure you get enough of it from rich sources. For example, you can eat two boiled eggs, yogurt, a cup of kefir, or a protein shake. Avoid beef and pork. Some raw nuts should also give you a caloric boost, for example, pistachios, almonds, Brazil nuts, and walnuts.

3. Avoid refined foods and carbs – Eliminate grains, sugar, potatoes, refined oil, and refined

starch. Keeping your carbohydrate intake low forces your body to burn your excess fat stores.

4. Time your workouts – If you are going to engage in intense exercise, try to schedule it toward the end of your under-eating phase. If your training regimen is very intense, you can consider eating a small protein-based meal before your workout.

Warrior Diet Sample Eating Plan

Daytime eating:

- Mornings – 2 glasses of water; or coffee or tea with no sugar; or whey protein

- Mid mornings – Fresh fruit or green veggie juice

- Lunch – Salad comprising tomatoes, onions, mixed greens, mushroom, cucumber, peppers, and sprouts; or poached egg

- Afternoon snack – Fresh fruit

Dinner/Main meal:

1. Raw veggies – Salad greens comprising any yellow, orange and red vegetables. Add broccoli sprouts if available. Salad dressing mixture of hemp, sesame, vinaigrette, and olive oil.

2. Cooked veggies – Steamed broccoli or cauliflower with mushrooms and onions.

3. Protein – Six ounces of chicken breast or some eggs topped with organic cheese.

4. Raw nuts and seeds

Fat Loss Forever Method

Now, if you thought the Warrior Diet is extreme, you are going to find this method of intermittent fasting to be very interesting. Consider this to be a combination of the best elements of the Warrior Diet, Eat-Stop-Eat, and Leangains. What makes the Fat Loss Forever method appealing is that it helps you lose fat AND allows you a "cheat" day to enjoy your favorite dishes.

So how does it work?

Well, you get a full 24 hours to eat whatever you desire, and then spend the next 36 hours on a total fast. No food whatsoever! You then split the remaining 4 ½ days of the week practicing the Leangains, Eat-Stop-Eat, and Warrior Diet.

If you find the Fat Loss Forever method confusing, don't worry. You are not alone. Most beginners have trouble keeping up with its schedule that requires you to interchange your fasting protocol every day. You must also have a high level of discipline to avoid overindulging on your certified cheat day.

The guys who designed this system knew it would be difficult to understand. This is why they recommend that you head over to their website so that they can assist you to develop a customized plan. Head over to

www.romanfitnesssystems.com.

Chapter 5

Intermittent Fasting and Exercise

If you usually take the time to exercise, you know that food provides fuel for your workouts. It is normal for you to be concerned about how fasting will affect your exercise routine.

The thing to note is that the timing of your eating and fasting will impact the effectiveness of your workout. But is it really risky to work out in a fasted state? And if so, what can you do to minimize that risk?

Are Exercise and Fasting Compatible?

If you are jogging, running, or lifting weights, your body mainly relies on glycogen (from stored carbs) to fuel your workout. The only time when your body doesn't depend on glycogen is when it has been depleted, and this only occurs when you are fasting. According to Dr. Pritchett, a sports dietetics specialist at the Central University of Washington, your body will then be forced to burn fat to produce energy. A study published in the *British Journal of Nutrition* reported that running before eating breakfast can help you burn 20 percent more fat compared to eating before going running.

Contrary to what most people believe, working out on an empty stomach can actually be beneficial. It is a well-known fact that Hugh Jackman practiced intermittent fasting to prepare for his role in the latest *Wolverine* movie. Did you notice how shredded he looked? Of course, that isn't what you are aiming for, but the point is that fasting can cut fat and still build muscle. This is primarily because of the flood of hormonal changes that help in fat burning and muscle building.

Two hormonal effects occur when fasting:

- Increase in insulin sensitivity – When you eat, your body releases the insulin hormone to help in the absorption of nutrients. The insulin then removes sugars from the bloodstream and stores them in the liver and muscles as glycogen, and also in fatty tissue. The problem is that we tend to eat too much too often, thus making our bodies resistant to insulin. Low insulin sensitivity may lead to cancer and heart disease, but it also makes it more difficult to lose body fat. By fasting regularly, the body releases insulin less often, thus making you more sensitive to it. When you add exercise to fasting, you ultimately make fat loss and muscle gain much easier.

- Increase in Growth Hormone (GH) – Fasting boosts the levels of GH in women by 1,300 percent. GH is known to cut body fat, boost muscle gain, and improve bone quality. Exercising while in a fasted state boosts production of GH, thus turbo-charging your fat loss and toning your muscle.

Now, it is important to note that other studies indicate some concerns. Some research shows that exercising in a fasted state causes the breakdown of muscle. If you exercise without eating some carbs, your body may begin to burn protein after a few hours.   Clearly, this will affect your performance, whether you are lifting weights or are doing some cardio. Coincidentally, it may be very difficult for you to power through a strenuous workout when your stomach is constantly growling.

However, if you go back to what we learned in the previous chapter on intermittent fasting techniques (especially the Leangains Protocol), you will notice that it is recommended you consume some BCAAs (Branched chain amino acids) right before your workouts. This will provide the necessary protein and energy to avoid muscle breakdown. Another recommendation we talked about was exercising about one or two hours before your fasting window ends. This means that you will soon eat something to provide fuel for your body.

Working Smart When Fasting

You really shouldn't worry too much about exercising while fasting. There are ways to structure your workouts such that you lose fat and prevent any other negative side effects. Here are a few tips to help you out when exercising and fasting:

1. Maintain a low intensity when fasting

The best way to gauge the intensity of your workout is through your breathing. If you are doing cardio when fasting, make sure that you are still able to have a conversation fairly easily. If you cannot, then you are probably working out too intensely and need to slow down. A light run or exercising on the elliptical probably won't leave you out of breath. The important thing is that you learn to pay attention to your body and stop working out the moment you feel dizzy. Keep a low intensity and don't push yourself.

2. Increase the intensity after you have eaten

The Leangains Protocol is very strict with how you schedule your meals and workouts. This is why it is a very effective way to lose fat while still maintaining your energy. The general rule is that if you want to work out after your fasting window is over, make sure that it is a high-intensity exercise. You have broken your fast, so there is enough glycogen to fuel your workout.

3. Engorge on high-protein meals

If you happen to be interested in building some serious muscle while fasting (yes, some women do want to gain muscle), make sure that you eat a lot of protein before and after lifting weights. The pre-workout meal will provide fuel while the post-workout meal is critical for helping your body repair and grow muscles. When practicing intermittent fasting, the important thing is to time your strenuous weight-lifting exercises between meals or snacks.

4. Snack within your feasting window

Your feasting window isn't just for eating meals; you can also snack if you want to. If you happen to be susceptible to low blood sugar, make sure that you snack on something two hours before you start working out. This will provide the energy necessary to push through your strength-training exercises. Go for a meal containing some fast-acting carbs and protein, for example, toast with peanut butter and slices of banana.

The reality is that different people may not have the same experience when exercising while fasting. Some people will report an improvement in performance while others won't. Nobody can tell you what time to work out when fasting and what to eat. However, the science behind it is clear, so the best thing is to try it out for yourself and see what works for you.

Chapter 6

Safety Tips for Women

Intermittent fasting has become more of a global health phenomenon, and research keeps revealing its inherent benefits to the human body. However, due to the fact that it impacts women differently, it is important to consider some of the things you need to watch out for.

As a woman, you cannot run away from the fact that you are biologically created to reproduce. Your body is always trying to create a hospitable environment for bearing a child, and this is only possible by keeping a tight leash on your hormones and accumulating fat. This is why your body is very sensitive to any kind of starvation signal. If your body detects any hunger pangs caused by lack of feeding for an extended period of time, it releases the hunger hormone *Ghrelin*. It won't be long before you find yourself craving to eat everything in front of you. It is this kind of reaction that causes many women to have an immense craving to eat during fasting, or binge eat once the fasting period is over.

Whenever your body senses some kind of starvation, it triggers a chain reaction. You suddenly become hyper alert and wakeful, and your memory and cognition receive a boost. This is your body's way of improving your chances of finding food quickly. Your body also resorts to the drastic measure of switching off any biological processes it deems unnecessary. One of these processes is menstruation. If you don't have enough calories to live, there is no need to try to support a pregnancy anyway. The process of shutting down your menstrual cycle comes via hormonal changes. This explains why most women will experience mood swings, longer or shorter menstrual periods, or even spotting.

So where are we going with all this?

Well, the truth is that such hormonal disruptions negatively impact your body. Intermittent fasting can disrupt your estrogen levels if you do not follow the right steps. The estrogen hormone is vital for a lot of processes, including bone formation and maintenance. It is clear to see how an imbalance in estrogen levels could lead you to end up with weak bones. Subsequently, you could be at risk of osteoporosis and bone breakages. The worst thing about it is that once your hormones are disrupted, it becomes extremely difficult to reverse the damage.

As a woman who is looking to lose fat and live a healthier life through intermittent fasting, you need to learn how to do it safely so that you avoid all the negative consequences.

Here are some tips that you need to keep in mind when practicing intermittent fasting:

1. Start gradually

You need to ease yourself into the new eating regimen by fasting for 10 - 12 hours every second or third day. Don't just dive into it as if it's an all-

or-nothing affair. Women experience better results when they start slowly, so spend the first one month gradually adapting your body to burning fat. For example, you can fast for 10 – 12 hours on Monday and Friday and see how you feel about that. Once you get the hang of it, you can then add more fasting days to your week.

2. Pay attention to your hormones

Your hormones are the biggest risk you take with intermittent fasting. Women's hormones play a sensitive role every 28 days. There are times when a slight change in diet, mindset, or stress level can result in hormonal imbalance, which may lead to future health issues. You should also monitor your thyroid and cortisol hormones, especially if you have suffered from adrenal fatigue or thyroid problems in the past. It is also recommended that you check the condition of your hormones before you start fasting. If you have a hormonal imbalance, don't fast. If you want to test your monthly hormone cycle and daily cortisol rhythm, you can use a salivary collection.

3. Avoid the urge to diet while fasting

Did you know that one of the biggest reasons why intermittent fasting fails to work for women is because they diet AND fast simultaneously? Intermittent fasting is not a diet! You cannot go on an intermittent fast and then start dieting within your feeding window. When your fasting window closes, that is your cue to start eating. Do not try to put yourself in a huge calorie deficit. When it's time to eat, consume a lot of calorie-dense, nutrient-rich foods. Never fast and diet at the same time!

4. Try to emphasize consumption of fats

If you want to prevent your body going into a huge calorie deficit, make sure that you eat a lot of healthy and nutrient-dense fats. Great sources of such fats would be free-range animals, nuts, eggs, unsweetened coconut oil, avocado, avocado oil, pasture-raised butter, olive oil, and olives. If you start making these foods part of your staple diet, you are guaranteed adequate calories and nutrients.

Another benefit of a high-fat diet is a reduction in stress levels during fasting. When you lower your carbohydrate intake and raise your fat consumption, you enhance the stability of your blood sugar. The problem with eating too many carbs is that your blood sugar levels become erratic, quickly rising up and then dropping a few hours later. This lack of glucose then triggers the release of the stress hormone, cortisol. With fats, your blood sugar is more like small waves rather than large peaks and valleys. There won't be any glucose to worry about, and you will have eliminated the stress response.

5. Avoid intense workouts

Try to exercise moderately for the first few weeks of your intermittent fasting. When your body has adjusted to the fasting state, you will begin to experience an improvement in your workouts. The most important thing, as described before, is to avoid placing undue stress on your body until it adapts to burning fat for energy. Your moderate exercises can begin with walking and then transition to short sessions of sprinting, jumping rope, and lifting weights.

6. Try not to obsess over losing fat

This may sound contrary to what this book aims to teach you, but there is a good reason to follow this advice. Yes, there are a lot of people who have managed to lose fat and get great-looking bodies through intermittent fasting. However, don't focus on using intermittent fasting solely to lose fat and become skinny. This may cause you to obsess over your body and use food to manipulate it.

So, what does this mean? It is better to think of intermittent fasting as a therapeutic way of attaining greater health benefits. Identify a deeper purpose for wanting to change the way your body looks. Are you suffering from brain fog or have problems maintaining your concentration? Intermittent fasting can help you improve brain health. Do you want to live longer and age gracefully? Intermittent fasting is known to slow down aging. Are you looking for a way to regulate your cardiovascular and blood lipid markers? Intermittent fasting can do that without using any pills.

7. Stop fasting if you start to feel bad

You are the one who knows yourself best, so if you begin to feel dizzy, tired, or weak, break your fast and eat. Intermittent fasting isn't for everybody, so always listen to what your body is telling you.

Chapter 7

Tips to Stay Motivated

Motivation or lack thereof plays a major role in your ability to stick to any diet. Intermittent fasting is no different. The normal tendency for most people is to start fasting with a serious motivation to change the way their body looks. However, as time goes by and they fail to see the results they were expecting, their inner drive starts to falter.

It is important to understand that nothing changes overnight. If there is a diet that promises you instant results, it is probably unnatural and not good for your body in the long term. Time is a factor in losing fat, and you have to make the commitment to keep going even when the first few weeks of fasting and exercise don't yield the expected results.

The truth is that week one, and two don't always show the fat loss. Some people even gain a bit of weight during this period! Just know that this is a possibility and perfectly normal. By the time you get to week three and four, you will definitely see some consistency in your fat loss.

So, what can you do when you feel you are in a slump and not seeing tangible results? Here are some ways to keep your motivation levels high:

1. Replace the scale with a mirror – Before you start your intermittent fast, stand in front of your mirror naked after a shower. Look at those areas of your body where you want to cut some fat and tone some muscle. You should take a "before" picture of what your body looks like so that you will be able to compare as the weeks go by. Keep this picture in a place where you will see it every day and use it to motivate you. You shouldn't rely on a scale because there are times when you will lose fat and gain some muscle tone, but your weight won't budge as expected. Lean muscle has replaced the body fat you have lost, so you may discover that your weight isn't

dropping as fast as you want it to. So, avoid using the scale to judge your progress and use the mirror instead.

2. Find a fasting buddy – It is easier to keep going when you know there is someone else fasting with you. It can be your husband, best friend, or family member. Sit down with them and walk them through the basics of the intermittent fasting technique you have chosen. Use each other as support on those days when one of you doesn't feel like fasting or exercising. It will be more fun when you have someone who you can plan meals with, shop for food with, train with and learn with. If you have someone else who is invested in your success, you won't want to do anything to let them down.

3. Use others for inspiration – While getting a fasting buddy is awesome, it's even better to find a community of people who have already used intermittent fasting successfully. You can research YouTube videos about others who

transformed their lives through intermittent fasting. There are also books and articles that can inspire you. There is also the option of joining Facebook groups and online forums. You will need others to support and encourage you when your motivation starts slumping.

4. Set achievable goals – It is best to start with short-term goals that you know you can achieve. Once you attain that goal, reward yourself, but don't do it with junk food. Get a massage or buy some new workout clothes. This will help boost your momentum and motivation.

5. Eat a variety of foods – You do not have to eat the same meals every day. This is boring and would kill any motivation you have. Find some interesting recipes made from the best foods recommended for fasting. This book has already given you some great meals in Chapter 4. Make sure that you eat healthy foods during your eating window. Exchange recipes with

your fasting buddy or search the internet for some low-calorie foods. Keep mixing things up and modifying your meals to create interesting meals.

6. Visualize what you will look like 6 to 12 months from now if you quit today – It's time to be brutally honest with yourself. When you feel your journey is getting too difficult (example: weight loss plateau), close your eyes and see your future self. You have quit fasting and have gone back to your old habits. What does your body look like? What does your life look like? You can either quit now and take the unhealthy route or focus on how many positive changes you have made so far. Think back to how you felt before you began fasting. You have made tremendous improvements to your life, both seen and unseen. Keep going!

7. Focus on how great you feel when fasting – Intermittent fasting can help you feel more energetic, creative, and focused. Use this

renewed alertness and euphoria to do things that you enjoy, whether personal or at work. Whenever you feel like giving up on your fast, remember how it makes you feel and how it is helping you achieve more in life.

8. Think of it as building self-control and discipline – Every day that you spend on a fast builds up your self-control and discipline. These are rare virtues in today's society, which is why many people struggle to do what it takes to succeed in life. You are choosing to pay the price today to achieve something greater tomorrow. The great thing about self-control and discipline is that these are muscles you can flex in other areas of your life. Your personal and professional life will benefit from having greater discipline and self-control. Even when you look in the mirror and fail to see any meaningful changes, just remember that you are getting stronger every day.

9. Focus on other benefits besides fat loss –
   Intermittent fasting has numerous other
   benefits apart from fat loss. Think about how
   you are benefiting from longevity,
   detoxification, improved brain health, blood
   sugar regulation, and much more. On those
   days when you feel down because you aren't
   seeing fat dropping off, focus on the other ways,
   you are benefitting.

10. Keep a progress journal – This is a great way to
    look at the positive changes you have been
    experiencing ever since you started your fast.
    Get a diary and start writing how you feel and
    all the progress you are making. It is important
    to take time to look at how your body and life is
    transforming. Look at how your clothes fit, the
    energy you now have to play with your kids, and
    the way your sleep has improved. Track your
    positive progress and whip out that journal
    whenever you feel yourself losing motivation.

11. Don't beat yourself up – Yes, there are days when you will fail and succumb to temptation. Things will get rough, and you will grab a cookie and start munching away. Be compassionate with yourself. Don't start talking negatively about yourself just because you didn't do things right. The important thing is to get back up and keep going.

12. **Pray and meditate** – When you start to feel discouraged, take some time to feed and strengthen your soul and spirit. Pray, read scriptures, and meditate. This will help you love yourself despite the challenges you face in life.

You have the power to lose fat and get the body you want. But you have to take the time to plan well and stay motivated. In the end, the results will show, and you will be glad that you pressed on with the hard work!

Chapter 8

The Biggest Mistakes to Avoid

So far, we have learned a lot about intermittent fasting and how it affects women and the human body in general. However, there are some mistakes that many newbies make when they dive into intermittent fasting without a plan.

Here is a summary of some of the most common and costly mistakes that you need to avoid:

Continuing to Eat Crap Food

One of the most common complaints people make is that they are following the fasting technique but aren't seeing results. When asked about their nutrition, the answer always reveals the problem. They are still eating processed foods (chips, candy, cake, crackers, etc.) and drinking sweetened beverages (sweet teas and soda). You cannot fast, exercise hard, eat junk food, and still expect that you will lose fat and tone that butt. You must decide to throw away all the unhealthy stuff and go for whole and unprocessed foods. There will be cheat days when you can indulge in something decadent, but don't make that part of your intermittent fasting lifestyle.

Not Keeping Yourself Busy

You cannot spend the day fasting and sitting around doing nothing. Staying idle is the worst thing you can do because you will start thinking about food. Get up and do something to stay active, as long as it keeps you away from food.

You Set Goals Too High

If you are a newbie to intermittent fasting, make sure that you don't start off with only one meal a day. You may think that going in hard from the start will help you torch all that fat, but it doesn't work that way. You cannot go from eating four to six meals a day to surviving on a single meal. You will mess up your hormonal cycles, and the negative effects will outweigh any benefits you gain. Learn how to transition gradually, as described in the Crescendo Method in Chapter 3.

You Fear Going Hungry

It's perfectly normal to feel hungry, but you will not die just because you go for a couple of hours without food. Most people have this irrational and morbid fear of depriving themselves of food, believing that all their muscles will be gobbled up. This fear can tempt you to cheat during your fasting window. Do not be afraid of a bit of hunger.

You Spend Your Days Staring at the Clock

Most newbies will develop an obsession with the clock when fasting. They will count down the hours, minutes, and seconds until they can rush to the kitchen and start bingeing. On the other extreme end are people who are afraid of breaking the "rules," so they make sure that they fast until the last second of the fasting window is over. Intermittent fasting is not that hard or strict. You cannot spend the day worrying and wondering about the timeframes and schedules. If your entire life starts and ends with your next meal, you will drive yourself mad. Just relax and enjoy the ride.

Obsessing Over the Sum of the Parts

Intermittent fasting is like a complex and dynamic system. There are a lot of individual pieces that form a large system. It is useless getting fixated on one small piece and forgetting that there are many more important things to focus on. For example, some people may worry about whether adding a teaspoon of cream to their coffee while fasting will ruin their chances of losing fat. Others wonder whether the 16/8 method is better than the 5:2 Diet. However, there are other bigger concerns that you should be focusing on, for example, your food selection; your training regimen; eating the right portions according to your goals; consuming enough proteins and fats, and so on. The whole is always greater than the sum of the parts. Focus more on spending a portion of your day or week in a fasted state, and the rest of the time feeding normally. Leave the trivialities alone.

Other Books by Author

IIFYM: *The Ultimate Beginner's Guide to If It Fits Your Macros*

Intermittent Fasting: *The Art and Science of Intermittent Fasting*

Slow Cooker IIFYM Cookbook: *Over 51 Delicious Recipes for Flexible Dieting*

Resources

www.draxe.com

www.ncbi.nlm.nih.gov/pmc/articles/PMC3680567/

www.vibrant-living.ca

https://www.ncbi.nlm.nih.gov/pubmed/23382817

http://journals.plos.org/plosone/article?id=10.1371/journal.pone.0052416

https://biohackingentrepreneur.com/intermittent-fasting-for-women/

www.exepriencelife.com

www.dailyburn.com

www.greatist.com

www.antonymichal.com

Nair PM, Khawale PG. Role of therapeutic fasting in women's health: An overview. J Mid-life Health 2016; 7:61-4

https://breakingmuscle.com/healthy-eating/a-womans-guide-to-intermittent-fasting